The Love of a Heavenly Father

By Angie Lithgow

Table of Contents

Introduction

When Jesus taught his disciples how they should pray, his opening words were: "Our Father which art in heaven." This shows that Jesus not only sees the Almighty God as his own father, but he also sees God as a father to all who seek Him. The purpose of this book is to explore the different facets of the parent/child relationship with the hopes of gaining a better understanding of our own relationship with God, our Heavenly Father.

Jesus's decision to use the word "father" when addressing his prayer demonstrates that God is a personal being with whom we can have an intimate relationship. Not only is God attainable to each one of us, but He also desires a close relationship with us. He has gone to great lengths to provide a way for us to know Him, but we must also do our part. Like all relationships, it is a two-way street. It takes both parties making a focused effort to develop closeness to one another. God cannot have a relationship with us if we refuse to open our hearts to Him.

In the chapters ahead we are going to explore some of the roles of a parent and how they relate to our relationship with God as His children.

Chapter 1: Creator

As a parent, two of the most special and memorable days of my life include the births of my son and my daughter. I am still in awe at the miracle of childbirth. Seeing their faces for the first time and hearing their little voices will be forever planted in my mind. Even the way they smelled and felt has left a lasting impression on me. I played a role in their creation, and now they are people who will grow up and impact the lives of others. I knew from the moment I met them that my life would never be the same. With such joy, however, came great fear. I had never had so much to lose. Before having children, I knew I could always handle what lay ahead of me. If I made mistakes or bad choices, I would face the consequences and keep going. But now someone else depended on me. In that instant, everything changed.

I remember when my son, Giggs, first entered the world. They placed him in my arms, and it didn't feel real. He was finally here, and he was mine. He had a head full of hair and a look of wonder. He was perfect in my eyes. I didn't want him out of my sight. My heart grew that day with a love I had never known before. I remember questioning how I could ever love another child as much as I love this one. Two years later, I would have the answer to that question.

The day I gave birth to Beckam, my daughter, I studied every detail of her little face. Her eyes were open wide, and she would not stop staring at me. The sight of her smile was contagious, and it made me smile right back at her. She was perfect to me. I would watch her sleep in complete peace, trusting me with her every need. But I knew this would not last forever. I knew that the storms of life lay ahead of her, and one day she would face heartbreak.

In both cases I knew their eyes would someday be opened to an imperfect world, and they would have choices to make. There would come a day when I could no longer protect them, and they would feel pain.

There is nothing I can do to prevent it from coming, but there is one thing for certain. As long as I am alive, they will never have to face the storms alone. I will always be available as a place where they can regain their strength, receive encouragement, and be reminded of how much they are loved. I won't be able to shelter them forever, but they will never be alone in their battles.

As our creator, God makes that same promise to His children. "I will be a Father to you, and you will be my sons and daughters, says the Lord Almighty" (2 Cor. 6:18). He longs to be close to us and be a part of our daily lives. He finds joy in His creation and in our existence. Those who love Him and trust Him are never alone. "Fear not, for I am with you; be not dismayed, for I am your God; I will strengthen you, I will help you, I will uphold you with my righteous right hand" (Isa. 41:10). He does not promise that life will be easy or that we will never experience pain, but He does promise to be there with us. He is a source of strength and encouragement.

Women sometimes take pride in their roles as mothers because they often take credit for "making" the baby. We look at our child with a feeling of accomplishment and experience a special connection in having known the child before birth. In actuality, we have no control over our child's design. How much more does the true creator feel for us, His creation? "For you created my innermost being; you knit me together in my mother's womb" (Ps. 139:13). We can never know the depth of God's love for us.

When my children were very young, I would tuck them into bed each night. I would always tell them that I love them, and without hesitation one of them would reply, "I love you more!" The game would ensue with who could say it last and who could say it the loudest. The kids would giggle to no end at our nightly ritual, but I knew the truth. See, I have been both a parent and a child, and I have experienced both kinds of love. I can honestly say that I love my children more than they love me. I also know that they will never love me as much as I love them, and I am okay with that. I know they love me as deeply as they know how. They love me as much as their little hearts will let them, but it is not the same as a parent's love for a child. They won't know how much I love them until they have children of their own. I often think this is the way God, my Heavenly Father, feels about me. I love God, and I tell Him often. I love Him as much as I know how and as much as my earthly heart will let me. However, each time I tell God that I love Him, I imagine a voice from heaven replying, "I love you more," and somehow, I believe it.

A few weeks ago, I posted a picture on social media of my husband, Rory, and me. The picture was taken early in our dating years, and we look like young children. I was amazed at the number of comments I received saying that our son and daughter look just like us. Some people even said at first glance they thought it was a picture of Giggs and Beckam. I also have a picture in our home of Rory's father holding him in a swimming pool. Rory must have been about six years old. People constantly ask me where Rory and Giggs were when that picture was taken. They can't believe that Rory is the six-year-old in the picture. Rory is one of five boys, and they all share a close resemblance. He is regularly mistaken for one of his brothers.

Creation is such an amazing thing, and I love how we are often made to resemble our family members. Likewise, we are all made in the image of God our Father (Gen. 1: 26–27). He could have chosen to create us to look different from Him, such as He did with animals and other life forms, but He chose to make us in His own likeness. What an honor it is to be made in His image. I have heard it said that imitation is one of the greatest forms of flattery. When you spend time with someone, you often begin to talk like them or take on their mannerisms. I have seen boys who stood or walked like their fathers. I have heard girls talk and choose words like their mothers. We have no greater example to imitate than our Heavenly Father. The more time we spend with Him in prayer and scripture and worship, the more we begin to resemble Him, not only in physical form, but also with our lives. Just as we are often a reflection of our earthly parents, we should strive to reflect our Heavenly Father's image.

Psalm 139

Of David.

¹You have searched me, LORD,
    and you know me.
²You know when I sit and when I rise;
    you perceive my thoughts from afar.
³You discern my going out and my lying down;
    you are familiar with all my ways.
⁴Before a word is on my tongue
    you, LORD, know it completely.
⁵You hem me in behind and before,
    and you lay your hand upon me.
⁶Such knowledge is too wonderful for me,
    too lofty for me to attain.

⁷ Where can I go from your Spirit?
    Where can I flee from your presence?
⁸ If I go up to the heavens, you are there;
    if I make my bed in the depths, you
are there.
⁹ If I rise on the wings of the dawn,
    if I settle on the far side of the sea,
¹⁰ even there your hand will guide me,
    your right hand will hold me fast.
¹¹ If I say, "Surely the darkness will hide
me
    and the light become night around
me,"
¹² even the darkness will not be dark to
you;
    the night will shine like the day,
    for darkness is as light to you.

¹³ For you created my inmost being;
    you knit me together in my mother's
womb.
¹⁴ I praise you because I am fearfully and
wonderfully made;
    your works are wonderful,
    I know that full well.
¹⁵ My frame was not hidden from you

when I was made in the secret place,
    when I was woven together in the
depths of the earth.
16 Your eyes saw my unformed body;
    all the days ordained for me were
written in your book
    before one of them came to be.
17 How precious to me are your thoughts,
God!
    How vast is the sum of them!
18 Were I to count them,
    they would outnumber the grains of
sand—
    when I awake, I am still with you.

Chapter 2: Protector

Before we had children, my husband had always been a heavy sleeper. He would sleep through thunderstorms, barking dogs, garbage trucks, and sometimes even the alarm clock. I never had to tiptoe around in the mornings or worry about turning on the lights. If he did not have to be up, he could sleep right through it. This all changed once he became a father. The slightest "peep" from the baby would send him to his feet. If the baby sneezed, coughed, or even sighed, he would immediately jump from bed to check on the baby. He would even hear noises that I didn't hear.

It didn't take long for us to figure out that we were not the type of parents who could sleep with the baby in our room. Even the slightest sound from the baby would wake us. We soon moved the baby into the nursery and kept the monitor close to the bed. We turned the monitor to a volume that drowned out the baby's normal sleeping sounds and only woke us when it was necessary. We slept much better, and it allowed us to be better parents the next day.

Our Heavenly Father also hears our cries. He hears our slightest sighs to our deepest sobs. And often when we cry out to Him, He responds in an instant. Psalm 121:3 says, "He who watches over you will not slumber." It is so comforting to know that He is standing watch over me, protecting me as a father does a child. One of my favorite Bible verses is Isaiah 58:9, "Then you will call, and the Lord will answer; you will cry for help, and he will say: Here am I." He not only hears me when I cry out in times of trouble, but He is also faithful when I cry out in times of repentance.

Kids often see their fathers as being big and strong. They see them as indestructible. They say things like, "My dad is bigger and stronger than your dad." When I was a kid, my brother and I thought our dad was huge. He seemed so big and powerful. We used him as a measuring stick to describe other things. My brother would always say things like, "He is bigger than Dad!" And to us that meant big! Now that my brother and I are adults, we laugh about it. So does my dad, who is only 5'9" and not the grizzly person we remember. Well, our Heavenly Father is all-powerful. He is bigger and stronger than anyone else's dad. He can calm the storm and close the mouth of a lion, and He protects His children.

One summer Rory and I took the kids to Africa to go on a safari. Rory is from South Africa, so it is always exciting to visit his family. The place we stayed was a private game reserve where we were assigned a tracker and a guide. We would go for game rides in the open-air Range Rover, which meant the vehicle did not have doors or a roof. I found this alarming. We were told that as long as we didn't stand up, the animals would not see us as individuals. They saw the vehicle as one being. They knew it was not food or prey, so they mostly ignored it in search of those things.

I was amazed at how close we would pull up to dangerous animals. Lions, cheetahs, leopards, etc. It was terrifying. I was also extremely concerned that the driver would stop the vehicle in open fields and let us out to "stretch our legs." They called the stops "drink breaks." The riders would get out, and the driver and tracker would prepare drinks and snacks for us. It was also the chosen time to use the restroom, which consisted of the closest shrub. They were so comfortable with the ritual that it didn't even faze them. I, however, was never comfortable with it. I would usually stay in the vehicle, and I would ask the kids to stay close, properly fulfilling my role as the over-protective mother.

On the last morning of our visit, we pulled into a valley for our final drink break. I stayed seated in the vehicle and watched as the rest of the group milled around the area. The kids were a little farther away than I preferred. They were kicking around in the dirt and playing. I still thought to myself to yell over the group for them to come back to the vehicle, but they were enjoying the break from riding. All of a sudden, I saw a lioness charging down the path toward the children. My heart stopped. I screamed, "Lion!" and everyone ran toward the rover. As the lioness charged toward the children, she suddenly stopped dead in her tracks. She began to growl at them with a growl that vibrated the vehicle. She stood still, growling three times at them while they took the opportunity to run toward the vehicle. Once they reached safety, she turned and headed back up the hill.

We were all stunned and shaken, to say the least. Even the rangers could not explain her behavior to let the children go unharmed. If a lioness feels threatened enough to charge into a group, then there is most likely going to be a victim. There is no explanation for her to stop and change her mind. I played the scenario over and over in my mind. It haunted me for days, and I rarely thought of anything else. I kept seeing the lioness charge my children and hearing her angry growl. I had trouble sleeping or even relaxing with the disbelief of what I had witnessed.

On the third night, as I lay in bed replaying the scene again in my head, my Heavenly Father showed me something. He showed me an angel standing in front of the children. The angel was male, and he stood confidently in the lion's path. She slammed on her brakes and growled at him, but he would not let her pass. Once the kids were safely in the vehicle, the angel was gone and the lioness returned up the hill. After seeing that, there was not a doubt in my mind that the Lord had protected those children. What a blessing to know that He is our personal protector. He can shut the mouths of lions, and He is a present help in our time of need. His power and protection have no limits.

The next day my son was talking about the lioness. I took the opportunity to tell him what the Lord had shown me. My son looked at me and said, "Mom, God showed me that same thing." I still stand in awe of our powerful Father's unfailing love and mercy. I am reminded of David and how he must have felt in his heart as he wrote Psalm 27. He faced much danger in his life and had many enemies. Still he found peace and assurance knowing he was a child of God. He trusted in God's protection.

Psalm 27

Of David.

1 The LORD is my light and my salvation—
  whom shall I fear?
The LORD is the stronghold of my life—
  of whom shall I be afraid?

2 When the wicked advance against me
  to devour me,
it is my enemies and my foes
  who will stumble and fall.
3 Though an army besiege me,
  my heart will not fear;
though war break out against me,
  even then I will be confident.

4 One thing I ask from the LORD,
  this only do I seek:

that I may dwell in the house of the LORD
    all the days of my life,
to gaze on the beauty of the LORD
    and to seek him in his temple.
5 For in the day of trouble
    he will keep me safe in his dwelling;
he will hide me in the shelter of his
sacred tent
    and set me high upon a rock.

6 Then my head will be exalted
    above the enemies who surround me;
at his sacred tent I will sacrifice with
shouts of joy;
    I will sing and make music to the LORD.

7 Hear my voice when I call, LORD;
    be merciful to me and answer me.
8 My heart says of you, "Seek his face!"
    Your face, LORD, I will seek.
9 Do not hide your face from me,
    do not turn your servant away in
anger;
    you have been my helper.
Do not reject me or forsake me,
    God my Savior.
10 Though my father and mother forsake

me,
   the LORD will receive me.
¹¹ Teach me your way, LORD;
   lead me in a straight path
   because of my oppressors.
¹² Do not turn me over to the desire of my foes,
   for false witnesses rise up against me,
   spouting malicious accusations.

¹³ I remain confident of this:
   I will see the goodness of the LORD
   in the land of the living.
¹⁴ Wait for the LORD;
   be strong and take heart
   and wait for the LORD.

Chapter 3: Provider

When our children were born, I felt the need to leave the workplace and stay home to care for them. I was blessed with a situation where this was an option, even though giving up my income would be a sacrifice. I was surprised to see that becoming a parent had the opposite effect on my husband. Suddenly he felt the need to work harder to provide even more for our growing family. I saw the additional responsibility he put on himself to give us what we needed and fill the role as the sole provider. He had additional mouths to feed and little bodies to clothe. He wanted to give the kids their heart's desires even if it meant we had to give up many of the comforts we had been used to before having children.

When I think back to my own childhood, I remember my parents being the same way. They rarely purchased anything for themselves, especially if my brother or I wanted the latest pair of shoes or a new ball glove. They sacrificed a great deal to provide us with the things we needed and, more often than not, the things we wanted. It brought them great joy to give us those things, and it brings my husband and me great joy to do the same for our children.

I believe God our Father also takes great joy in providing for His children. He loves to bless us not only with the things we need but also the things we desire, especially when what we desire is in line with His will for our lives. The thing we should desire most is a relationship with Him. Psalm 37:4 says, "Take delight in the Lord, and he will give you the desires of your heart."

In Matthew 7:9–11, Jesus reminds us that our Heavenly Father wants to bless His children by saying, "Which of you, if your son asks for bread, will give him a stone? Or if he asks for a fish, will give him a snake? If you then, though you are evil, know how to give good gifts to your children, how much more will your Father in heaven give good gifts to those who ask Him?"

Once the kids were older, I went back into the workforce. My boss and I usually meet several days a week before the start of our workday. It is a way for us to address work-related issues before stepping into the busy office of buzzing emails and ringing phones. During that time, we also talk about other things of interest. I found myself talking quite a bit about the Israelites. I know that seems odd, but at that time I was studying their customs and cultures and loved sharing what I was learning.

My boss, being a fellow believer, would ask me about my studies. A few weeks after my study had ended, my boss sat down to breakfast and presented me with a huge surprise. He said he had heard me mention that it would be my dream to go to Israel. He had attended church that Sunday, and his church was arranging to take a group on a pilgrimage to Israel. He had signed me up and paid for me to go. Even more, he was giving me an additional two weeks of vacation time to use for my trip. I couldn't believe it. It is still hard for me to believe today. I went on the trip of a lifetime traveling to all parts of Israel. The knowledge I gained, the things I saw, and the emotions I felt while I was there will never be forgotten. I am so thankful for such a generous boss, but I am also so thankful for a Heavenly Father who I have no doubt orchestrated the whole thing. He knew how much I desired to learn more about Him and His people and His Son, and He provided me with the gift that allowed me to do that. What a wonderful provider!

When I was a very young child, one of the first sets of Bible verses that I set to memory was the 23rd Psalm (The Lord is my shepherd . . .). Those six verses have remained embedded in my memory for most of my life, and they paint a wonderful example of what I would consider the perfect provider. Shepherds care for their flock's daily needs. They live among their sheep and protect them from danger. They love their sheep, and they are even willing to lay down their lives for their sheep. A shepherd knows his sheep and can tell when one is missing from the flock. He will go seek out the lost sheep to bring it back into the fold. In turn, the sheep know their shepherd. Sheep tend to wander, but they respond when they hear their shepherd's voice. They follow their shepherd because they trust the path on which he leads them. They cannot protect themselves, so they place their full dependence on their shepherd. It is such a beautiful picture of trust and provision.

While I was in Israel, I was able to travel through the areas where David worked as a shepherd before he became a king. I could imagine him writing many of the psalms on the very land where we were. We witnessed shepherds and sheep still feeding on the same hillsides that David tended. We visited the shepherd's fields in Bethlehem where the angel appeared to announce the birth of the Savior. The King James Version of Psalm 23 that I had learned as a child played over and over again in my mind.

Psalm 23

Of David.

¹The Lᴏʀᴅ is my shepherd; I shall not want.

² He maketh me to lie down in green pastures: he leadeth me beside the still waters.

³ He restoreth my soul: he leadeth me in the paths of righteousness for his name's sake.

⁴ Yea, though I walk through the valley of the shadow of death, I will fear no evil: for thou art with me; thy rod and thy staff they comfort me.

⁵ Thou preparest a table before me in the presence of mine enemies: thou anointest my head with oil; my cup runneth over.

⁶ Surely goodness and mercy shall follow me all the days of my life: and I will dwell in the house of the Lᴏʀᴅ forever.

Chapter 4: Teacher

If I knew in advance that I would not be around to raise my children, what would I do to ensure they knew that I loved them? How would I impact their lives and decisions without being physically present? How could I teach them the things I would want them to know? What would I tell them about myself, or how would I explain to them ways to deal with decisions they will face in their lives? I would write it down.

When my children were born, I started a journal to each of them. I would write things in their journals that I would want them to know and understand in case I wasn't around to tell them. I know it sounds morbid, but it brought me peace to know they would have my words for a later reference. They could always pick up my journal if they wanted to be reminded of my love for them or get my advice on something that I wanted to share.

It later dawned on me that God provided the same thing for us, His children. When I am doubting myself, or I need sound advice, or I just want to hear my Heavenly Father's voice, I pick up my Bible. It reminds me of God's love for me and guides my decisions. Psalm 119:105 says, "Your word is a lamp for my feet, a light for my path." Reading God's word gives me direction and makes me feel closer to Him.

As children of God, studying God's word helps us grow in our relationship with Him. We start to learn more about Him, and we are better able to recognize His will and leading. We gain a better understanding of who He is. As a result, we have a better chance of distinguishing His voice from that of the world. If we aren't reading God's word and hearing what He teaches, we are missing out on a closer relationship with Him. He wants to teach us. He wants us to learn from Him, much in the same way an earthly father would. He has wisdom to share, and He has provided it to us in His word. We should desire to know more about Him and make spending time with Him a priority.

When I first met my husband, Rory, I was immediately intrigued by him. I wanted to know everything I could about him. I wanted to know about his past, where he came from, his family, his friends, his interests. We didn't have Google back then or even Facebook, so I couldn't just "stalk" him online. It took some effort and it took time, but I was happy to invest both to learn more about him. Things naturally progressed and the learning process continued. We have been married for over twenty years, and I am still learning things about him that I never knew. And I hope there is always more to learn.

By spending time together, the relationship has grown. It has strengthened and matured. Much in the same way, spending time with God in prayer and reading His word helps us grow and mature in our knowledge and relationship with Him. We find our decisions becoming influenced by wanting to please Him and make Him proud, and our desire grows to be more holy and pleasing in His eyes. This change is reflected in our actions, our thoughts, our words, and our lives.

When I was getting to know my husband, Rory, early in our dating process, I learned that he wasn't a Christian. He called himself a Christian, but he had never truly given his life to Christ as his savior. He would tell me that he was a decent person. He had never killed anyone, and he didn't steal. If there was a heaven, he would probably be there. He was twenty-five years old and had never needed anything more in his life. He was "fine," so I married him. I spent a lot of time in prayer asking God to touch Rory's heart, to show him the need for a savior and for forgiveness of sins. That opportunity came in an unexpected way.

We had been married three years when Rory noticed a lump on my breast. He became instantly concerned and unsettled, and he asked me to go see a doctor. The doctor sent me home with an eye roll saying I was only twenty-eight with no family history and nothing to worry about. They were going to have me return in six months to see if anything had changed. I was great with that response, but Rory wasn't. After three doctors sent me home with the same explanation, Rory scheduled an appointment with a surgeon for a biopsy. He wanted me to have the lump removed.

I went to the appointment on my own. As I was sitting in the exam room, I could hear a lady's voice. She was on the phone saying that she had a patient who had been examined and sent home by other doctors. She said it was her youngest patient yet, but she could tell by the ultrasound that the young girl had breast cancer. I listened intently as I wondered if she was talking about me. A few minutes later, it was confirmed. I had breast cancer. Hearing the news had little to no effect on me. I was at complete peace with it. I didn't have children at the time, and I was strong. Most importantly, I had faith. Faith that whatever the outcome, I would be okay. Rory, on the other hand, did not have that faith, and he was a mess.

On the day of my surgery, the doctor told Rory the procedure would take four hours. So, he waited. And waited. Four hours passed, then five, six, seven hours without a word. Rory broke down. He was afraid they had found so much cancer that I wouldn't survive the surgery. He knew in his heart where I would spend eternity, but he realized that he wasn't sure about himself. He got down on his knees in the hospital waiting room and cried out to God. Through tears, he asked for forgiveness and turned all his faith and trust over to Christ.

When I woke up in recovery, Rory stood over me a changed man. I could see the change on his face, but I wasn't sure what had happened. Rory told me about the long wait and his anxiety turning to fear and brokenness and leading him to seek God. I couldn't believe it. We were both praising God in the recovery room when my surgeon finally spoke up. She was confused. She said she had sent two nurses to inform Rory on the delay. She was angry that neither nurse had done as they were told.

She said she had performed the surgery in four hours, as usual. She was leaving the operating room when she stopped dead in her tracks. She was overwhelmed with the feeling that she had not taken enough tissue. She said the feeling was so strong, she couldn't continue. She called anesthesiology back in and canceled her next appointment. She performed the procedure all over again, taking extra tissue until she knew she had done all she could.

Rory and I both knew the real reason the nurses never showed up with the information. God was at work, and we were grateful for the extra time and the disobedient nurses.

Once Rory began to study the Bible for the first time, he realized how much there was to learn. He wasn't sure where to start. I recommended that he teach the first-grade Sunday School class at our church. After all, the kids weren't old enough to embarrass him, and he could study and learn the Bible stories alongside of them. Much to my surprise, he agreed. I'll never forget one Sunday morning seeing Rory coming down the hall with a strange look on his face. "Really?" he said. "A fish swallowed a man and then spit him back out? Is that one of those parable things, or did that really happen?"

When I told him that really happened, he just shook his head. After that, he made reading God's word a priority, and he still does. It was important to Rory for us to bring our children up to know the Bible. So, after our children came along, we decided to enroll them in a Christian school. The Bible teacher at their school was very committed and taught the kids so much. At times, I thought he went a little too deep in his lessons with these small children, but I was wrong.

When my son, Giggs, was in the third grade, my daughter, Beckam, was in kindergarten. Beckam was taking gymnastic lessons after school, and that always gave Giggs and me time to sit and talk. I remember one afternoon when Giggs seemed a little down. He wasn't quite himself, and I could tell something was bothering him. I asked what it was, and he began to explain. He said, "Mom, you know David in the Bible?" I replied that I did. Then he asked if I knew the story of David and Bathsheba, which I did. He then went on to ask if I knew how Nathan the prophet confronted David with the story of the man and his only lamb. I became more intrigued as Giggs went into great detail about how it really bothered him that David took Uriah's only beloved wife much like the rich man that took his poor neighbor's only beloved lamb.

Giggs was visibly upset with David's decision and finished by saying, "What David did was very wrong." I agreed with Giggs and asked if he had learned that in Bible class that day. Much to my surprise he said, "No, I learned it in the first grade, but I just now understood it." My heart sank. God's words had been at work in Giggs's little heart for three years, but they were not forgotten.

They were waiting for the proper moment to make an impact on him.

I was reminded that God's word is living and speaks to me at just the right time. My Heavenly Father plants His words in my heart and brings them to my attention as He sees fit. However, I am responsible for reading the words He has provided. Isaiah 55:11 says, "So is my word that goes out from my mouth: It will not return to me empty but will accomplish what I desire and achieve the purpose for which I sent it." God's teaching does not return void. It accomplishes His purpose. 2 Timothy 3:16 says, "All Scripture is God-breathed and is useful for teaching, rebuking, correcting and training in righteousness." So many things we read and hear go in one ear and out the other. That is not so with God's word. Every teaching He has provided to His children has an objective and will achieve His purpose.

Psalm 25

Of David.

1 In you, LORD my God,
    I put my trust.

2 I trust in you;
    do not let me be put to shame,
    nor let my enemies triumph over me.
3 No one who hopes in you
    will ever be put to shame,
but shame will come on those
    who are treacherous without cause.

4 Show me your ways, LORD,
    teach me your paths.
5 Guide me in your truth and teach me,
    for you are God my Savior,
    and my hope is in you all day long.
6 Remember, LORD, your great mercy and
love,
    for they are from of old.
7 Do not remember the sins of my youth
    and my rebellious ways;
according to your love remember me,
    for you, LORD, are good.

⁸ Good and upright is the LORD;
    therefore he instructs sinners in his
ways.
⁹ He guides the humble in what is right
    and teaches them his way.
¹⁰ All the ways of the LORD are loving and
faithful
    toward those who keep the demands of
his covenant.
¹¹ For the sake of your name, LORD,
    forgive my iniquity, though it is great.

¹² Who, then, are those who fear the
LORD?
    He will instruct them in the ways they
should choose.
¹³ They will spend their days in prosperity,
    and their descendants will inherit the
land.
¹⁴ The LORD confides in those who fear
him;
    he makes his covenant known to them.
¹⁵ My eyes are ever on the LORD,
    for only he will release my feet from
the snare.

¹⁶ Turn to me and be gracious to me,
   for I am lonely and afflicted.
¹⁷ Relieve the troubles of my heart
   and free me from my anguish.
¹⁸ Look on my affliction and my distress
   and take away all my sins.
¹⁹ See how numerous are my enemies
   and how fiercely they hate me!

²⁰ Guard my life and rescue me;
   do not let me be put to shame,
   for I take refuge in you.
²¹ May integrity and uprightness protect me,
   because my hope, LORD, is in you.

²² Deliver Israel, O God,
   from all their troubles!

Chapter 5: Disciplinarian

Growing up, my dad was the disciplinarian in our household. My brother and I both knew our dad had a narrow set of rules. Oftentimes Dad wouldn't even have to say a word to change our behavior. I remember sitting in church with my brother and getting tickled about something. The giggling would begin, and we knew it was going to be a problem. We would turn our heads down the pew to see Dad's serious glare looking back at us. We knew that meant we had better pull it together or else we would have to face the consequences.

Our mom was not much on behavioral discipline. Her rules and louder volumes were usually reserved for keeping us away from the hot stove or watching out for oncoming traffic. If our behavior became a problem, Mom preferred to threaten us with telling our father as opposed to dishing out any real punishment. That was usually all it took to get the response she wanted.

During those early childhood years, my brother and I obeyed our parents mostly out of fear for getting in trouble. We preferred to avoid the punishment that we knew followed the disobedient behavior. As we got older, our obedience to our parents was more out of respect and trusting their guidance and rules. Now that I am a parent, I have a much better understanding of the need for discipline. Dad was trying to teach us to be respectful and exhibit self-control. Mom's rules were more focused on everyday protection and trying to keep us safe. Both areas of discipline are necessary to create healthy, productive young adults.

When I see children who lack any discipline, I have a hard time not chalking it up to lazy parenting. It is much easier to remain seated on the couch and allow your child to do as they please than to actually get up and redirect the child's behavior for the benefit of everyone. As an adult, I am grateful that I had parents who cared enough to discipline me in a loving but effective way.

Our Heavenly Father has also established rules and laws for the benefit of His children. He doesn't just require obedience to prove that He is in charge or to rule with a heavy hand. His rules have a purpose. Some of them were created to keep His children safe and protected, while others are required to develop mutual respect, love for each other, and self-control. God's laws are always for our benefit. From the beginning, God established a set of rules for His people to follow. Some of the rules limited the things they could eat or how they ate them. These rules kept His children safe from becoming sick and focused on their health. Other rules prevented social behaviors that brought harm to one another. These laws taught His children respect and self-control.

To enforce rules, discipline is required. Healthy levels of fear, respect, and trust must be established, or the rules are ineffective. I am glad I have a Heavenly Father who cares enough to establish rules and discipline and carry them out in a loving way for the benefit of His children.

I knew when I made the decision to have children that I would not be giving birth to little robots who would obey my every command. Even though I was responsible for their existence, they would still have a will of their own. The best I could hope for was to have a positive influence on them and guide them in the ways they should go. This is no small task.

Our Heavenly Father could have created us to do His will no matter what. He could have taken away our ability to disobey Him and replaced it with controls to make sure we did what He wanted us to do. However, He chose to give us free will. He created us to think on our own and make our own decisions. He gave us the freedom to choose our own direction. With that freedom comes great responsibility. Our Heavenly Father provides His children with His spirit, His guidance, His influence, but He does not impose His will on us. It is up to us to choose obedience to Him or disobey His perfect will for us.

When my children deliberately disobey me, it is disappointing. It hurts to think that they chose their own conflicting behavior knowing that I would disapprove. It makes me wonder about their love, trust, and respect for me. However, I must allow them to learn and grow from choosing their own actions. They will need to learn for themselves to endure the consequences of their decisions. In John 14:21, Jesus said, "Whoever has my commands and keeps them is the one who loves me." There is a connection between love and obedience. A parent doesn't want a child to show love merely by professing it.

The saying "actions speak louder than words" has great wisdom. One way a child can show love to a parent is through obedience. As a child of God, keeping His commandments can be seen as evidence of our love for Him. Doing His will above our own, denying ourselves without hesitation and complaining, is a reflection of our love and trust for Him. David understood the importance of keeping his Father's commandments and honoring His covenant as displayed in his writing of Psalm 103.

Psalm 103

Of David.

¹ Praise the LORD, my soul;
   all my inmost being, praise his holy name.
² Praise the LORD, my soul,
   and forget not all his benefits—
³ who forgives all your sins
   and heals all your diseases,
⁴ who redeems your life from the pit
   and crowns you with love and compassion,
⁵ who satisfies your desires with good things
   so that your youth is renewed like the eagle's.

⁶ The LORD works righteousness
   and justice for all the oppressed.

⁷ He made known his ways to Moses,
   his deeds to the people of Israel:

8 The LORD is compassionate and gracious,
   slow to anger, abounding in love.
9 He will not always accuse,
   nor will he harbor his anger forever;
10 he does not treat us as our sins deserve
   or repay us according to our iniquities.
11 For as high as the heavens are above
the earth,
   so great is his love for those who fear
him;
12 as far as the east is from the west,
   so far has he removed our
transgressions from us.

13 As a father has compassion on his
children,
   so the LORD has compassion on those
who fear him;
14 for he knows how we are formed,
   he remembers that we are dust.
15 The life of mortals is like grass,
   they flourish like a flower of the field;
16 the wind blows over it and it is gone,
   and its place remembers it no more.
17 But from everlasting to everlasting
   the LORD's love is with those who fear

him,
  and his righteousness with their
children's children—
¹⁸ with those who keep his covenant
  and remember to obey his precepts.

¹⁹ The LORD has established his throne in
heaven,
  and his kingdom rules over all.

²⁰ Praise the LORD, you his angels,
  you mighty ones who do his bidding,
  who obey his word.
²¹ Praise the LORD, all his heavenly hosts,
  you his servants who do his will.
²² Praise the LORD, all his works
  everywhere in his dominion.

Praise the LORD, my soul.

Chapter 6: Forgiver

My husband, Rory, is very good at apologizing. He finds it easy to accept any blame that needs placing. Even when it is not his fault, he is quick to say he is sorry. He says the words "I'm sorry" more times in one day than I say in a year. Rory is from South Africa, so he apologizes with an accent. "I'm sorey," he will say. The first time I met him was in a restaurant where he was ordering a glass of water just a couple of feet from where I was seated. Receiving his order, he turned too quickly, losing control of his drink. The entire glass of water ended up in my lap. All I could hear was his voice saying, "Sorey, sorey, I'm so sorey."

Now, I know spilling water is an accident. He didn't choose to drench me. I was never mad at him for it, and apologizing in that type of situation is easy. However, what about when I do something that I know is wrong— even worse, when I choose to do it. I, unlike my husband, find it very difficult to apologize. Even when I know it is my fault, those words don't come easy. When I apologize for something, I really mean it. I am mournful over it. I was raised in a home where I didn't hear a lot of apologies. It wasn't because no one ever did anything wrong. We just didn't say we were sorry for what we did wrong. So, when I met Rory, I couldn't understand how easy it was for him.

My daughter is much the same way as my husband. She is quick to apologize, especially if she thinks it will defuse the situation. She will tell me she is sorry before I can even finish telling her why I am upset with her. She apologizes often, and sometimes I wonder if she means it. I find her apologizing for the same things over and over and over again. Is she really sorry? If she is truly sorry, why does she keep doing it? It usually has something to do with picking her clothes up off the bathroom floor. Day after day she is sorry for leaving them there.

One evening I asked Beckam to "come pick her clothes up off the ba—" She was apologizing before I could finish my sentence. I thought to myself, "I don't want another apology. I just want you to stop doing it." At that moment, I thought how God must feel the same way about us. Sometimes I feel as if I commit the same sins over and over and over. I ask God for forgiveness, and I know He forgives me, but why don't I just change my behavior? Why don't I just stop committing the sin?

I can't imagine what it must have been like for the Israelites. They were required to make sacrifices for the forgiveness of sins. The blood of an innocent animal was required. I think if a blood sacrifice was required for my sinful behavior, it would make me think twice before choosing to sin. Sometimes I wonder if I take advantage of the ease at which I can receive forgiveness. I know it would be better if I would just be obedient from the beginning. 1 Samuel 15:22 says, "But Samuel replied: Does the LORD delight in burnt offerings and sacrifices as much as in obeying the LORD? To obey is better than sacrifice, and to heed is better than the fat of rams." I am reminded that forgiveness for my sin did require innocent blood. It required the very precious blood of an innocent man, the Son of God, Jesus. My Heavenly Father would rather that I just obey instead of seeking forgiveness. It is popular in today's society to say, "It's easier to ask for forgiveness than to ask for permission." But if we know it is going to require seeking forgiveness, maybe we shouldn't want permission to do it.

By contrast, nothing touches me more than when one of my children sincerely apologizes for something they did. When I see the tears and feel the emotion they are experiencing, there is no way I can continue to express anger against them. I truly do forgive them and can't keep myself from wrapping them in my arms as I accept their apology. I imagine God feeling the same way about our sincere, heartfelt, mournful apologies. He knows our hearts, and He is a forgiving Father. He does not hold our trespasses against us when we bring them to Him.

Psalm 32

Of David.

¹ Blessed is the one
  whose transgressions are forgiven,
  whose sins are covered.
² Blessed is the one
  whose sin the Lᴏʀᴅ does not count
against them
  and in whose spirit is no deceit.

³ When I kept silent,
  my bones wasted away
  through my groaning all day long.
⁴ For day and night
  your hand was heavy on me;
my strength was sapped
  as in the heat of summer.

⁵ Then I acknowledged my sin to you
  and did not cover up my iniquity.
I said, "I will confess
  my transgressions to the Lᴏʀᴅ."
And you forgave
  the guilt of my sin.

⁶Therefore let all the faithful pray to you
    while you may be found;
surely the rising of the mighty waters
    will not reach them.
⁷You are my hiding place;
    you will protect me from trouble
    and surround me with songs of
deliverance.

⁸I will instruct you and teach you in the
way you should go;
    I will counsel you with my loving eye
on you.
⁹Do not be like the horse or the mule,
    which have no understanding
but must be controlled by bit and bridle
    or they will not come to you.
¹⁰Many are the woes of the wicked,
    but the LORD's unfailing love
    surrounds the one who trusts in him.

¹¹Rejoice in the LORD and be glad, you
righteous;
    sing, all you who are upright in heart!

Chapter 7: Sacrifice

I cannot imagine what it would be like to lose a child. As a parent, losing a child is my greatest fear. I have seen the suffering in the eyes of parents who have lost a child. I am aware that they have felt emotions I have never felt. It becomes a part of them they can never escape. Even when they appear to be going on with their daily lives, it never leaves them. I don't think a parent can ever truly recover from such a tragic loss. Today as I sit down to write, it just happens to be Passover. As soon as I climbed out of bed this morning, I began to think about the life that was tragically given for me. I think about the sadness that my Heavenly Father must have felt as His beloved son took his final breaths. I know we often think about the sacrifice Jesus made for us, and we should never forget that, but for now let's consider the sacrifice God made as a parent of this child.

Having two children, I am very aware of how different they are from each other. They think differently, they act differently, and I often wonder how they could have come from the same set of parents. Even though they are different they are both so incredible in my eyes, and I love each of them with the same amount of love. If one of them committed an awful crime and was required to pay for the crime with their life, I can't imagine how devastating that would be. Even worse, what if their death meant that they would have to spend eternity in a place of constant agony and separation from me? I would never again be able to see their face, comfort them, protect them, or have a relationship with them. I don't know how I could cope with life knowing what lay ahead for my child.

What if the only way I could save that child from eternal separation would be to ask my other child to suffer a torturous death in exchange for both of them to spend eternity with me in a glorious paradise? How could I even ask that of my innocent child? How could I ask the blameless child to pay the price for the deserving child? How could I allow my underserving child to face torture and death when I knew I had the power to stop it?

To complicate matters worse, God had to choose to ask a perfect child, one without sin or blame, to suffer for a child whose life was filled with sinful choices and selfish decisions. He had to choose to sacrifice a child who was faultless and undeserving of punishment to be tortured in exchange for a child who committed evil deeds and was deserving of death. How could He allow Jesus, His obedient and loving son, to die for me, a disobedient child with a life full of sin? What an incredible, compassionate decision of love that my Heavenly Father made on my behalf. We do not deserve salvation based on our actions and choices. Jesus did not deserve death based on his sinless life. However, our God was willing to turn His blameless son over to the cruel hands of man to beat him, mock him, nail him to a cross, and die an undeserving death because of His love for us, His children. He allowed this to happen so that we would not have to spend eternity separated from Him. That is how much He loves us.

I have a brother who is two years younger than me. We were never really close growing up, and much of that was my fault. We were very different people, and honestly, I didn't give him much time or affection. As we grew into adults, our relationship began to change. I started to see him differently, and I realized that we didn't have to be similar to be close. I have grown to love my brother, and I know he loves me. I am always amazed at the stories of siblings who donate a kidney to a brother or sister or risk their life in some other way for a family member. How can you ever repay someone for such a generous gift? It makes me wonder how Jesus could ever choose to give his life for mine. I also think about my two children. Would my son be willing to sacrifice in such a way for my daughter? Would she do the same for him? Would one be willing to give their own life for the other if they knew it could change their eternal destination?

When I think about Jesus, sometimes it is hard for me to remember that he was a man who faced the same challenges that we face in everyday life. He was given the free will to make his own choices, and he was not forced into obedience. Jesus had to deal with earthly temptations and rely on God's word and prayer to give him strength and wisdom just like we do. He buried himself in God's teachings and made his relationship with God the top priority of his life. He must have known what lay ahead, but it didn't stop him from continuing on in God's will.

In the Garden of Gethsemane, Jesus knew he would soon be faced with the toughest decision of his life. He separated himself from the others to be alone with God in prayer, and he prayed with every ounce of energy he had. He was seeking the strength and courage to continue on the path of God's will. He was not being forced to hand his life over. Ultimately, it was his decision to make. He took the judgment on himself and paid the price that was required for our sins.

Several years ago, I read a fable about a flock of geese written by an unknown author. Whenever I see a flock of birds in the sky, I recall the story. It tells about a farmer who refused to believe in Jesus because he didn't believe that God would come to us in human form. One night a snowy blizzard swept across his land, and he could hear loud thumping noises outside. When he looked out, he saw a flock of geese caught in the storm. They were unable to fly in the strong winds and kept hitting into the side of his barn. He felt sadness for them and wanted to help. He thought if he could get them to fly into the barn, they would be safe and warm and would survive the storm.

He went out into the weather and opened the barn doors for them, hoping they would fly inside. Instead, they panicked and scattered in all directions. He tried many things to get them to understand and go into the barn, but nothing worked. Worried for their lives, he began to ask himself how he could possibly save them. If only he could become one of them, and he could lead them into the safety of the barn. Maybe then they would follow him and live. At that moment, the farmer understood God's heart toward us and fell to his knees in worship.

The story reminds me of God's compassion for us and His desire for us to follow Him so that we can be saved and live life in its fullness. He was even willing to send His Son, Jesus, to us to provide the way.

Psalm 51

Of David.

1 Have mercy on me, O God,
   according to your unfailing love;
according to your great compassion
   blot out my transgressions.
2 Wash away all my iniquity
   and cleanse me from my sin.

3 For I know my transgressions,
   and my sin is always before me.
4 Against you, you only, have I sinned
   and done what is evil in your sight;

so you are right in your verdict
and justified when you judge.
⁵Surely I was sinful at birth,
sinful from the time my mother
conceived me.
⁶Yet you desired faithfulness even in the
womb;
you taught me wisdom in that secret
place.

⁷Cleanse me with hyssop, and I will be
clean;
wash me, and I will be whiter than
snow.
⁸Let me hear joy and gladness;
let the bones you have crushed rejoice.
⁹Hide your face from my sins
and blot out all my iniquity.

¹⁰Create in me a pure heart, O God,
and renew a steadfast spirit within me.
¹¹Do not cast me from your presence
or take your Holy Spirit from me.
¹²Restore to me the joy of your salvation
and grant me a willing spirit, to sustain
me.

¹³ Then I will teach transgressors your ways,
   so that sinners will turn back to you.
¹⁴ Deliver me from the guilt of bloodshed, O God,
   you who are God my Savior,
   and my tongue will sing of your righteousness.
¹⁵ Open my lips, Lord,
   and my mouth will declare your praise.
¹⁶ You do not delight in sacrifice, or I would bring it;
   you do not take pleasure in burnt offerings.
¹⁷ My sacrifice, O God, is a broken spirit;
   a broken and contrite heart
   you, God, will not despise.

¹⁸ May it please you to prosper Zion,
   to build up the walls of Jerusalem.
¹⁹ Then you will delight in the sacrifices of the righteous,
   in burnt offerings offered whole;
   then bulls will be offered on your altar.

Chapter 8: Inheritance

One of my favorite things about being a parent is being able to bless my children. Nothing fills my heart more than giving them something that brings them joy. Seeing the looks on their faces as they open a gift or their reactions of excitement about what they received is something that thrills me. I think I get this enthusiasm from my dad. Growing up, Dad always loved to give us gifts. Maybe part of it was because both of my parents worked very hard for everything we had. We didn't receive gifts throughout the year, but they always made sure we had something to open on our birthdays and at Christmas.

As soon as the gift was purchased, my dad could hardly contain himself. He would constantly bring it up in his teasing high-pitched tone that "somebody has a birthday coming up" or "I wonder what Santa is bringing this year." Sometimes he would offer up little hints to try to get us to show excitement about the possibility of receiving what they had picked out. My mom would always have to step in to make sure he didn't take it too far. "Now, Danny" is all she would have to say, and he would let it rest. To this day he still does it even though we are adults, though to a much lesser extent. He loves to give gifts to those he loves.

Giving is so much more than spending money on someone. Some of my favorite things that I have ever received or given are not high-dollar items. Sometimes they cost nothing more than time. Giving is a way to show appreciation or affection for others without the expectation of anything in return. It is a loving gesture that shows you were thinking of someone else and that you value them. As Christians, the Bible is clear that we are called to give generously and sacrificially.

Two of the greatest gifts we could ever receive were given to us by our Heavenly Father. He gave us His Son, Jesus, who provided the way for salvation through the forgiveness of our sins. He also gave us the gift of the Holy Spirit to be our advocate and to counsel us for the rest of our days. It is the presence of the Holy Spirit that assures believers that we are children of God and is described as the guarantee of our inheritance (Eph. 1:13–14). In 1 Peter 1:4–5, Peter describes this inheritance as one "that can never perish, spoil, or fade. This inheritance is kept in heaven for you, who through faith are shielded by God's power until the coming of the salvation that is ready to be revealed in the last time."

An inheritance is such a special gift. It usually isn't something we have earned but instead is handed down to us from someone who came before us and loved us. What an amazing feeling it must be to know you can provide your children with something of value that may help make their lives easier or give them freedom from worry or need long after you are gone.

Before my mom passed away, she was able to get all her affairs in order. She made handwritten notes and attached them to different things that she possessed so that my brother and I would know their origin and what they meant to her. She and my dad decided that the house they acquired together would be passed down to my brother and I as an inheritance. It brought her great comfort to know she was leaving something of value behind for us. One of the last conversations I had with my mom was her telling me about their decision. She said she would never have to worry about my brother and I having a place to live because the house would be ours. I could see what that meant to her and the importance it held. Hopefully one day my husband and I will be able to do the same for our children.

When I think about the inheritance that awaits us from our Heavenly Father, I cannot begin to imagine what is in store. Much like an earthly inheritance, it is a matter of grace and not earned. It reminds me of the story of the prodigal son found in Luke 15:11–32. A father has two sons, and the younger one asks for his inheritance. The father obliges and gives the young son his portion of the estate. The young son leaves the father and squanders all that he was given. After he is hungry and destitute, he remembers his father. He decides to return home and seek forgiveness from his father and plans out what he will say by making three statements: [18b]'Father, I have sinned against heaven and against you. [19]I am no longer worthy to be called your son; make me like one of your hired servants.' [20]So he got up and went to his father.

"But while he was still a long way off, his father saw him and was filled with compassion for him; he ran to his son, threw his arms around him and kissed him." This image is so touching to me. His father had been waiting and watching for him to return with anticipation. During this time, it would not have been acceptable for a dignified man to run. Men usually wore long garments and sandals, and running was not easy or proper. It showed a tremendous sense of urgency. He must have been so eager to restore the relationship that His heart was overflowing.

[21]"The son said to him, 'Father, I have sinned against heaven and against you. I am no longer worthy to be called your son." At this point, the father did not even give him a chance to make the third statement he had prepared. Instead, the father's first word was "Quick." He couldn't wait another second to make amends, to offer forgiveness, and to bring his son back into the right state of son and heir.

I believe that our Heavenly Father feels the same way about us. Whenever we desert Him, turn away from Him, treat him as if He was dead, I believe it grieves His heart. He doesn't just write us off. He is patient with us as He waits and watches with anticipation for our return. He longs for us to come back home. And when we do show true repentance and humility and return to Him, He does not delay making us right with Him once again. He has compassion for us and quickly changes our condition and our standing with Him. He brings us back into the fold with rejoicing.

[22]"But the father said to his servants, 'Quick! Bring the best robe and put it on him. Put a ring on his finger and sandals on his feet. [23]Bring the fattened calf and kill it. Let's have a feast and celebrate. [24]For this son of mine was dead and is alive again; he was lost and is found.' So, they began to celebrate."

This prodigal son was prepared to return home as a slave, but instead his father completely restores him back into the full privilege of being his son. That is what our Heavenly Father does for us. Romans 8:16–17 describes Christians as being adopted sons of God, and therefore "heirs of God and co-heirs with Christ." What a glorious inheritance that awaits God's children, which He has promised to those who love Him.

Psalm 16

Of David.

¹Keep me safe, my God,
　　for in you I take refuge.

²I say to the LORD, "You are my Lord;
　　apart from you I have no good thing."
³I say of the holy people who are in the
land,
　　"They are the noble ones in whom is all
my delight."
⁴Those who run after other gods will
suffer more and more.
　　I will not pour out libations of blood to
such gods
　　or take up their names on my lips.

⁵LORD, you alone are my portion and my
cup;
　　you make my lot secure.
⁶The boundary lines have fallen for me in
pleasant places;
　　surely I have a delightful inheritance.
⁷I will praise the LORD, who counsels me;
　　even at night my heart instructs me.

⁸I keep my eyes always on the Lord.
   With him at my right hand, I will not
be shaken.

⁹Therefore my heart is glad and my
tongue rejoices;
   my body also will rest secure,
¹⁰because you will not abandon me to the
realm of the dead,
   nor will you let your faithful one see
decay.
¹¹You make known to me the path of life;
   you will fill me with joy in your
presence,
   with eternal pleasures at your right
hand.

Conclusion

I realize that many people are not as fortunate as I am to have a loving earthly father; this does not exclude anyone, however, from seeking God as their Heavenly Father. John 1:12 says, "Yet to all who did receive him, to those who believed in his name, he gave the right to become children of God."

No matter how wonderful our earthly fathers are, our Heavenly Father is so much greater. We should never limit our understanding of fatherhood to our own fathers, no matter how good or bad they are. All earthly fathers have sinned, have weaknesses, limitations, and shortcomings, but our Heavenly Father has none of these things. 1 John 3:1 says, "See what great love the Father has lavished on us, that we should be called children of God! And that is what we are!"